A DARTNELL HIGH-PERFORMANCE

GETTING THE BEST OF STRESS

How to Use Pressure to Improve Your Performance

FEATURING

Built-In Learning Reinforcement Tools

Case Studies

Personal Productivity Exercises

Customized Action Plans

Individualized Pre- and Post-Session Skill Assessments

COVER ILLUSTRATION: RANDALL ENOS

DARTNELL is a publisher serving the world of business with books, manuals, newsletters and bulletins, and training materials for executives, managers, supervisors, salespeople, financial officers, personnel executives, and office employees. Dartnell also produces management and sales training videos and audiocassettes, publishes many useful business forms, and many of its materials and films are available in languages other than English. Dartnell, established in 1917, serves the world's business community. For details, catalogs, and product information write:

THE DARTNELL CORPORATION
4660 N. Ravenswood Avenue
Chicago, IL 60640-4595, U.S.A.
Or phone (800) 621-5463 in U.S. and Canada
www.dartnellcorp.com

ISBN #0-85013-343-2
Library of Congress #98-073532

CONTENTS

5 Humor & Crisis: The Light and Dark Sides of Stress

INTRODUCTION

Stress is a part of life. It always has been. It always will be. It is not a "modern" development that has grown with the technological age. Our prehistoric ancestors experienced it. Whether their stress came from the tension of stalking a saber-toothed tiger or from an argument with a mate, they too felt the forces of stress playing upon their lives. So has every generation since.

We are much more aware of stress today, however, owing in large part to the tremendous amount of material devoted to its study. By now almost everyone is familiar with "stress" in its broad strokes and has also heard the advice for countering or reducing it: physical activity, taking some time off, managing reactions to it, and developing outside interests. Like taking an aspirin for a headache, these measures are, generally speaking, widely known and effective.

While we have duly noted these measures in this workbook, we wanted to move beyond them. We wanted to present simple and specific strategies for dealing with stress that apply to stresses encountered in the workplace — stresses with causes such as individual work overloads, conflicts with internal and external customers, and unrealistic or unclear responsibilities and goals. *Getting the* **Best** *of* **Stress** features strategies, techniques, and tips to deal with each of those areas and more.

Along the way you will discover a great deal about stress itself — what it is and isn't — and discover that some of the things you thought you knew about stress are not true. You will discover the part you play in creating and adding to the stress in your own life. And you will learn methods for reducing your stress level rather than increasing it.

Getting the **Best** *of* **Stress** is not a psychological cure-all for every stress that besets you. It is, rather, a guide to reducing stress in the work-related situations you are most likely to deal with on a frequent basis. We think you will find it informative, practical, useful, and occasionally entertaining. Don't hesitate to have a little fun as you learn ways of *Getting the* **Best** *of* **Stress**.

1

How Stress Begins

INTRODUCTION

Stress in the workplace has to come from somewhere, doesn't it? It can't simply be an all-pervasive force that seeps into everyone's job, wreaking havoc along the way. It is caused by *something,* isn't it?

Well, yes and no. Stress on the job does have its origins and causes. Unfortunately, though, those origins and causes, like stress itself, can come from almost everywhere. Including from within ourselves.

On the brighter side, being aware of how and why stress occurs is a major first step toward keeping it under control. That, happily enough, is the subject of Session 1, **How Stress Begins.**

As in all five of the sessions in this workbook, we'll begin with a *Pre-Session Skill Level Assessment*. This is a series of statements on which you'll be asked to rate your abilities. It will provide a benchmark to measure how much you'll progress by the end of the session.

Our first article goes right to the heart of the matter. *The Sources of Stress* clues you in to the real, sometimes behind-the-scenes reasons why you're running into stressful situations. It's backed up by an exercise to help you quickly distinguish between a long-term stressful environment on the job and stressful situations. That one's titled *Particular Stressors vs. Constant Stress.*

Next comes *A Quick Check-on-Your-Stress Test*, a little quiz to see how good your stress-handling skills are right now.

Then we'll turn our attention to how you can be a source of the problem yourself in *Three Ways You Put More Stress on Yourself*, which is what makes up Parts I, II, and III of *I Shoulda, Hadda, Oughta Done That.* In it you'll discover ways in which you almost unthinkingly add to your own stress level practically every day. (You'll also learn how to stop doing it.)

After pointing out some of the *Warning Signs of Stress*, we'll move on to our *Case Study*, which is titled *Good News, Bad News*. It revolves around a stress-related topic that has become all too familiar in the workplace in recent years.

The *Answers Section* is next, in which we'll give replies and suggested solutions to the various exercises included in this session. *Do You Remember?* is a little feature designed as a pop quiz to see how much you recall from the session. So be alert.

Finally, we'll feature a *Post-Session Skill Level Assessment* in which you'll get another chance to rate your talents and an *Action Plan* designed to identify and improve your personal strengths and weaknesses in the area of stress reduction.

It all starts on the next page with **How Stress Begins.**

PRE-SESSION SKILL LEVEL ASSESSMENT

Using the chart below, rate your own skills as they relate to the following statements.

WEAK	AVERAGE	STRONG
1–4 points	5–7 points	8–10 points

I can recognize the physical warning signs of too much stress.	________
I know how to avoid putting more stress on myself.	________
I am aware of the dangers of negative thoughts.	________
I know the difference between a stress incident and prolonged stress.	________
I can identify sources of stress in my work environment.	________
I know how to identify the sources of stress.	________
I realize that being aware of sources of stress can help in dealing with it.	________
I am good at changing my "self-talk" in order to minimize stress.	________
I am able to control or minimize stress on a daily basis.	________
I am able to control or minimize stress overall.	________
TOTAL RATING	________

WEAK	FAIR	GOOD	STRONG
Under 40	41–55	56–74	75–100

A total score of 55 or less means there is room for improvement. A score between 56 and 74 means you are doing well but can do better. Any score over 75 means it is just a matter of building on your strengths.

THE SOURCES OF STRESS

What causes stress on the job? It's usually not too difficult to identify some of the particular sources at a given point in time. The boss yelled at us. There isn't enough time to do a particular project. Co-workers aren't pulling their weight and we have to cover for them. These kinds of stress-producing incidents — or stressors — happen all the time.

When stressors are not isolated or passing incidents, however, the real problems occur. Work-related stress often falls into categories, and the first step in dealing with them is to identify and recognize them. Here are some of the most common categories, or sources, of stress in the workplace:

1. Conflicts with superiors

2. Conflicts with co-workers

3. Ongoing workloads that are too heavy for one person to perform effectively

4. Confusion or lack of clarity about your job responsibilities or what your superior expects from you

5. Lack of direction; vague or unclear goals from upper management.

Can you think of any other stress sources such as these that are based upon your own experience at work? Write them down.

6. ____________________

7. ____________________

8. ____________________

Now think of a *particular incident* at work that you found stressful (for example, "the boss yelled at me"). Into which category (or categories) from the list above do you think this incident falls? Write it below.

____

____

____

____

PARTICULAR STRESSORS VS. CONSTANT STRESS

To manage your own stress level effectively, it is important to distinguish between the particular incidents of stress and the sources of stress that are chronic or ongoing.

Example: An angry customer chews you out.

If this is a rare incident, it is a particular stressor.

But, if your job is to deal with dissatisfied customers every day and this happens fairly frequently, it is a source of stress.

Why is it important to distinguish between the two? Because a particular incident — as bad or stressful as it may be — usually stands alone and should be dealt with as is. But if that incident is part of a larger pattern, if it has come about because it stems from a source, dealing with the incident alone will not remove the cause of the stress.

To deal with constant job-related stress, you must identify and try to deal with its source.

Look at the stressful incident you described on the preceding page and try to think of a few more. Are they related to a larger pattern, to one of the five sources of stress? If so, try to identify what the source of the stress really is. Then think of a strategy you can use to address the problem and write it below.

Notice that we said "address" the problem, instead of "solve" it. Often it is not possible to make the source of stress disappear completely, short of changing jobs. Nevertheless, there are ways to minimize the problem — many of which we'll be covering later in this workbook. For now, the important thing is to realize where that stress is coming from and to try to deal with it.

Sources of the stress: ______________________________

What I can do to address the source:

____

____

____

____

QUIZ

A Quick Check-on-Your-Stress Test

You have little control over irate callers and customers and the number of them that may come in at one time. But you *do* have control over how you react to the stress these situations create. Take the following quiz to see how well you respond to stress on the job. Answer each question **YES** or **NO**; then score yourself below.

	YES	NO
1. Do you take at least 15 minutes every day — during lunchtime or a break — to get some simple exercise, such as walking or stretching?	______	______
2. Do you take time at the start of your day to relax in a quiet, peaceful environment?	______	______
3. Do you take a few minutes at the end of your day to review the customer contacts or other efforts that were a success?	______	______
4. Do you watch your intake of caffeine and nicotine?	______	______
5. Do you plan realistic and attainable goals for the day and for the week?	______	______
6. Do you regard customer complaints as challenges rather than as problems?	______	______
7. Do you meet with colleagues to "blow off steam" and discuss common problems and frustrations, striving to maintain a good sense of humor?	______	______
8. Do you seek challenges outside the office, such as hobbies or volunteer work?	______	______
9. Do you spend time talking over your workday with a friend, a spouse, or other family members and listening to feedback?	______	______
10. Are you able to shrug off comments made in anger by customers or co-workers?	______	______
Total Number of **YES** Answers	____________	

SCORE YOURSELF: If you scored eight or more **YES** answers, you are handling stressful situations fairly well. You understand the importance of balance between your life at work and your personal life, and you have found outlets for your stress. A score of seven or less indicates you need to find ways to ease the tension you're experiencing at work. Study the questions in the quiz for ways you might begin easing the stress in your life. It's important that you learn how to manage stressful situations. Your health and your career may depend on it.

THREE WAYS YOU PUT MORE STRESS ON YOURSELF, OR I SHOULDA, HADDA, OUGHTA DONE THAT

Part I

Faced with a situation, we often make it more stressful for ourselves than it already is. We put more stress on ourselves than the situation calls for. And we do it so effortlessly that we are hardly aware of it. We simply think or say one of the following phrases to ourselves:

1. I should ...

2. I have to ...

3. I ought to ...

Have you ever stopped to realize how many times you say those words to yourself? Take a moment and think back to a time at work when you were under stress. What did you say to yourself when it first came up?

1. I should ______________________________

2. I have to ______________________________

3. I ought to ______________________________

These types of phrases, and this type of thinking, put more stress on you. They create an obligation for something you feel you "must" do, or a guilt for something you "should" have done. And that creates more stress.

Memorize these phrases. It's the only way you'll have a chance at forgetting to use them, or at least at modifying them, as you'll see in Part II.

Part II

Oh sure, it's easy to say to stop thinking in terms of "shoulds" and "ought tos" and "have tos." It's also easy to say "lose weight," "get in shape," or "don't think of a purple giraffe for the next two seconds."

The fact is, these thinking habits are ingrained and not at all easy to overcome. So let's not even try. Let's see if we can outsmart them and slowly change them. Just a little.

For instance, instead of *I should*, why not try a milder variation? Instead of …

1. I should rewrite that report before I give it to the boss.

How about …

1. Maybe I could rewrite that report before I give it to the boss.

A small, subtle change, but potentially an important one. It is no longer the stress of an obligation you are putting on yourself, it's an interesting possibility, an opportunity, or maybe even a challenge. Which of these feelings would you prefer?

Below, write five alternative ways to rephrase any of the inner statements that begin with *I should, I have to,* and *I ought to.* You will find some suggestions in the *Answers Section* on page 11.

1. ______________________________

2. ______________________________

3. ______________________________

4. ______________________________

5. ______________________________

I SHOULDA, HADDA, OUGHTA DONE THAT

Part III

The three statements we've been discussing in Parts I and II are not the only ways to put more stress on yourself — they are simply the most common.

There are many different ways to say (or think) them, and all have the same effect of putting additional stress on you. Think carefully for a few moments and try to recall other similar phrases, whether or not you usually use them. Write them below.

1. ______________________________

2. ______________________________

3. ______________________________

4. ______________________________

5. ______________________________

You'll find some of them listed in the *Answers Section* on page 11.

WARNING SIGNS OF STRESS

When we begin to experience too much stress at work, our bodies will usually warn us. There are many ways this stress can manifest itself, but among the most common physical symptoms to appear are

1. Backaches

2. Sweating or a feeling of being "overheated"

3. Headaches

4. Excessive fatigue

5. Queasy stomach

Try to remember these warning signs.

CASE STUDY: GOOD NEWS, BAD NEWS

The good news was that John had survived his company's final downsizing. The bad news was that he now had to do the work of two of his former co-workers who had been let go. And that was in addition to his own regular workload.

John worked in the customer relations department of a national distributor's regional office. He was responsible for handling questions and complaints on deliveries. Due to the volume of business his firm did, it was not uncommon for him to get a half dozen calls a day on items that were late or lost. His job was to track down the missing orders.

His new workload — he was now taking nearly 20 calls a day — was making it impossible for him to do the job in a timely fashion. Tracking down a lost order took time. The calls were backing up, and the customers were getting angry at him for not resolving their problems quickly.

After two weeks of this, John found himself fighting a tendency to become short and irritable with the customers. He was having trouble sleeping, and he arrived at work fatigued. And the problems kept getting worse.

What should John do? What would you do? Write your solution below. Some suggested approaches are in the *Answers Section* on page 12.

____

____

____

____

____

____

____

____

ANSWERS SECTION

FROM I SHOULDA, HADDA, OUGHTA DONE THAT, PART II

The key is to think in less self-demanding terms in order to put less pressure and stress on yourself. Also, certain ways of phrasing can actually make you view the issue with anticipation rather than worry or guilt. For example:

Instead of *I should, I have to,* or *I ought to,* try these phrases:

1. What if I took a stab at doing it again? That might impress them.

2. I could try taking another run at it.

3. It might be a good idea for me to ...

4. I think I'll consider doing ....

The specific words are less important than the way in which you say them to yourself. The objective is to avoid putting highly stress-producing thoughts in your mind.

FROM I SHOULDA, HADDA, OUGHTA DONE THAT, PART III

Other self-talk phrases that will put additional stress on you are

1. I'd better ...

2. I'd best ...

3. I guess I'm going to have to ...

4. I must ...

5. I've got to ...

FROM CASE STUDY: GOOD NEWS, BAD NEWS

The source of John's increasing stress is obviously his work overload. He can, and probably should, try various stress-reducing techniques to help him cope. They will help him control the stress and manage it better.

They will not, however, remove the stress. That has become inherent in the new job description (his handling three times the number of complaints he did before).

He has several options open to him. If he can control and adjust to the new stress level, he may choose to do nothing else. Or he may choose to discuss the matter with his supervisor. If he does, he will have to be careful how he approaches the matter. In the wake of the recent downsizing, the supervisor may simply tell him that if he can't handle the job, they'll find someone who will. Or the supervisor may be sympathetic but say there is nothing she can do.

John should point out the risk to the company of angering its customers and that it is in their best interest to give him some help. He must make it clear that he is doing all one person can do and that the problem is a function of time. No matter how many hours he puts in, he can't resolve all of the complaints quickly enough. He should also document his daily workload to illustrate the additional pressures and the customer disservice that has stemmed from his work overload.

He has two things going for him. First, he was kept on while others were let go, which may mean his superiors considered him to be the most highly skilled. Second, many downsizings are followed by organizational adjustments as the newly structured company goes through its version of a shakedown cruise. Not all problems can be foreseen, and it's possible that an intelligent management will realize there's a problem in John's area and give him some assistance.

Failing a change in his workload or a newly developed ability to handle the stress, John should begin to think about looking for another job.

DO YOU REMEMBER?

Here's our workbook version of a little pop quiz to see what you can recall from this session. Try to fill in the answers without looking back.

How many of the *Warning Signs of Stress* can you recall? Write them below.

1. ____________________

2. ____________________

3. ____________________

4. ____________________

5. ____________________

POST-SESSION SKILL LEVEL ASSESSMENT

Based on what you have learned in Session 1, rate yourself again on the following statements. When you are finished, compare your total score to the one you earned at the beginning of this session.

WEAK	AVERAGE	STRONG
1–4 points	5–7 points	8–10 points

I can recognize the physical warning signs of too much stress.	______
I know how to avoid putting more stress on myself.	______
I am aware of the dangers of negative thoughts.	______
I know the difference between a stress incident and prolonged stress.	______
I can identify sources of stress in my work environment.	______
I know how to identify the sources of stress.	______
I realize that being aware of sources of stress can help in dealing with it.	______
I am good at changing my "self-talk" in order to minimize stress.	______
I am able to control or minimize stress on a daily basis.	______
I am able to control or minimize stress overall.	______
TOTAL RATING	______

WEAK	FAIR	GOOD	STRONG
Under 40	41–55	56–74	75–100

A total score of 55 or less means there is room for improvement. A score between 56 and 74 means you are doing well but can do better. Any score over 75 means it is just a matter of building on your strengths.

ACTION PLAN

Many of the skills and techniques you have learned in this session are interrelated. Building on your strengths is a good place to start improving your overall abilities, but you can't afford to overlook your weaknesses either.

List below your three best scores (your strengths) and your three lowest scores (your weaknesses) from the ratings on the preceding page.

STRENGTHS	**WEAKNESSES**
1. ______________________	1. ______________________
2. ______________________	2. ______________________
3. ______________________	3. ______________________

Comparing the two lists, can you see any ways in which you can use your strengths to improve your weaknesses? If so, write them down.

____

____

____

____

____

Now reexamine your three biggest weaknesses. Since it's best to work on them one at a time, list them in order. Start with the one you think will be the easiest to improve upon, followed by a more difficult one, and then the most difficult one.

Next to each, set a timetable for concentrating on them (one week, two weeks, and so on):

WEAKNESSES	**TIMETABLE FOR WORKING ON IMPROVEMENT**
1. ______________________	1. ______________________
2. ______________________	2. ______________________
3. ______________________	3. ______________________

Using the ideas and information from this session, list at least one technique you can practice to improve each weakness.

1. ____

2. ____

3. ____

If you cannot determine a technique or course of action you think will be effective, talk to your supervisor about ideas that can be applied to your specific situation.

At the end of the time frame you set for improvement on *all* your weaknesses, look again at the *Post-Session Skill Level Assessment*. Rate yourself once more on all the statements listed. You will probably find improvement not only in your weak areas, but in the others as well.

SUMMARY

Stress is virtually everywhere. It's an all-pervasive fact of life. It can be good, bad, or something in between, depending to an extent upon our reaction to it.

Keeping that in mind, the main points to remember from this session are that stress has two major sources: external and internal. The external sources come from our environment. The internal sources come from within ourselves. It would seem that the internal stresses — those we put upon ourselves — would be far easier to control because we are in control of ourselves. But as you have seen, that is not necessarily the case.

Internal stress can be as difficult to manage as external, and both often require the effective use of stress management techniques such as those we have covered in this session. Try to master as many of them as you can — and watch your stress level decline.

Your Internal Response to Stress

INTRODUCTION

No two people are alike. This is especially true when it comes to dealing with stress on the job. Have you ever noticed how some people fret and worry when confronted with a situation, while others — faced with the same situation — take it in stride, like water rolling off a duck's back?

These reactions have to do with a principle you have probably heard stated a hundred times in one variation or another: "It's not so much the stressful situation itself as the way you perceive it," or "It is your reaction to the stressful incident that determines how much stress you feel." Yes, different people do react differently. The reasons for different reactions and how you can change your reactions to reduce stress is what Session 2, **Your Internal Response to Stress**, is all about.

Our internal response begins in our head with all the thoughts we are constantly thinking and all the things we are constantly telling ourselves. That's called "self-talk." Even though we are always doing it, we are often not aware of what we are saying.

We begin with our *Pre-Session Skill Level Assessment* on self-talk so you can get an idea of how aware you are of what you are thinking. The first article, *How Self-Talk Affects Us*, explains how this works and how it very often leads to our putting more stress on ourselves.

Am I My Own Worst Enemy? will give you practice in becoming more aware of this tendency and changing negative statements into positive ones.

The Alligator Technique is a simple little method for catching yourself before you stress yourself out, and *Leap Not to Conclusions* will show you exactly how you often do yourself in. To illustrate the point, we follow with *A Fun Exercise to See If You Can Drive Yourself Bonkers*, a lighthearted look at a very serious matter.

Our *Case Study: An Encounter in the Elevator* will give you a chance to put this newfound knowledge to work in aid of a young worker who is about to stress herself out over a very normal incident.

And lest we forget the physical, the next feature is a quiz titled *Actions Too Can Bring on a Positive Attitude*. There's more than one way to combat stress, and this test will give you a few more ideas.

Our *Answers Section* is next, followed by the *Do You Remember?* quiz, the *Post-Session Skill Level Assessment,* and the *Action Plan*. We think you'll find this exploration of your inner thoughts extremely interesting and useful in your daily contest with stress.

Here's Session 2, **Your Internal Response to Stress**.

PRE-SESSION SKILL LEVEL ASSESSMENT

Using the chart below, rate your own skills as they relate to the following statements.

WEAK	AVERAGE	STRONG
1–4 points	5–7 points	8–10 points

I have a good awareness of my own "self-talk."	_______
I understand the importance of self-talk and its effects on me.	_______
I know how to interrupt or stop negative self-talk.	_______
I know of different actions that can help develop a positive attitude.	_______
I recognize how negative thoughts can get out of control.	_______
I know methods for changing negative thoughts.	_______
I am good at not jumping to negative conclusions.	_______
I am good at not exaggerating a bad situation.	_______
I realize how I put stress on myself.	_______
I avoid excessive worrying about work.	_______
TOTAL RATING	_______

WEAK	FAIR	GOOD	STRONG
Under 40	41–55	56–74	75–100

A total score of 55 or less means there is room for improvement. A score between 56 and 74 means you are doing well but can do better. Any score over 75 means it is just a matter of building on your strengths.

HOW SELF-TALK AFFECTS US

"Self-talk" is nothing more than the thoughts and perceptions we have about what is happening around us and to us. It is the inner dialogue that we are constantly having with ourselves. It is our internal reaction, analysis, and judgment of what is happening. And to say it has a major affect on our feelings, attitudes, and outlook is to greatly understate the matter.

We touched upon this subject in Session 1 in the exercise *Three Ways You Put More Stress on Yourself.* That was an introduction to a topic that is key to controlling stress: self-talk.

How aware are you of your own self-talk? How much do you know about it? Have you ever stopped to consider how you think about things? Try the following exercise.

1. Your boss has just called a meeting for your department. At the meeting, she announces that your department is going to be reorganized. What do you think would be your first thought (the first self-talk words you say to yourself)? Write it down.

____

____

____

2. Your supervisor comes by and asks you to stop in his office for a minute. What is your first self-talk thought? Write it down. Then write the second thought you have.

____

____

____

____

3. At your performance review, your superior congratulates you on an above-average performance. She then urges you to do even better. What is your first thought?

____

____

____

Look over your self-talk replies. Generally, do you see a pattern? Were your self-replies mostly negative? Positive? Fearful? Confident? Suspicious? Excited? Hopeful? What else?

Write how you would describe them.

____

____

____

____

If you can detect a pattern, you may get a clue to how your self-talk colors your outlook on your job, your career, and yourself. Try to become more aware of your self-talk and how it affects you.

AM I MY OWN WORST ENEMY?

In the short run, there is often little or nothing you can do to prevent a stressful incident from occurring. You can't dictate an easier workload to the boss. You can't stop an angry customer from calling you. You can't extend an impossibly short deadline. But, when the uncomfortable occasion confronts you, you can help to determine how much stress you actually experience by monitoring and changing your self-talk.

Take the following example:

You are fairly new at your job. Your supervisor calls you in and asks you to do an analysis of a problem that has been hurting the company. He wants you to suggest alternative approaches and he needs the report in a week.

You quickly see that a week is barely enough time, even if you were familiar with the problem. Being new at the company, you only have the vaguest idea of what's involved and will have to spend a considerable amount of time just learning what the trouble is. You mention that fact, but your manager brushes it aside, saying that it won't take long to get up to speed on it and that he's looking for fresh thinking on the problem. As you leave his office, your first thoughts are

1. He's got to be an idiot to think I can get this done in a week. He should know that isn't possible. Why is he doing this to me?

2. If I don't come up with the solution, he'll think I'm dumb. How am I supposed to solve the problem when no one else has so far?

3. If I don't do a great job on this I'm done for. I'll be back on the street looking for another job in no time.

There's obviously a great deal of negative self-talk here, and it's adding more stress to an already stressful situation. You are becoming your own worst enemy, and now you have to fight both your deadline and yourself.

Before trying to change these reactions, however, analyze them and try to determine where the distortion in this type of thinking lies.

What would you say is incorrect about the thinking in statement 1? Is it an accurate assessment of the situation? Or is it a distorted one? If so, how? Write your ideas below.

____

____

____

____

Do the same for statement 2.

____

____

____

____

Do the same for statement 3.

____

____

____

____

Answers are in the *Answers Section* on page 29.

Now write three reactions that would represent positive self-talk if you were in the situation in the example. Don't necessarily try to rewrite or change the three statements. Instead, just give three examples of positive self-talk statements you could make to counteract the negative self-talk.

1. ____

____

2. ____

____

3. ____

____

Some suggested replies are in the *Answers Section* on page 29.

THE ALLIGATOR TECHNIQUE

The two preceding exercises have provided an idea of how your self-talk affects you and shown you some ways you can begin to change it. While change is not easy, with time, practice, and repetition it can be done. The hardest part, however, is catching yourself in the act of indulging in that negative, stress-increasing self-talk.

Thoughts come and go with lightning speed. An entire sequence of thoughts can flow through our minds in seconds. We talk to ourselves so fast and so constantly that often we are barely aware of what we are thinking. In the meantime we have colored our attitudes and outlook and have piled a great deal of unneeded stress on ourselves — almost before we know what we are doing.

The crucial step in stopping negative self-talk is to catch ourselves doing it. This is not an easy task when you've been accustomed to thinking a certain way. You will need something a little outrageous to serve as a warning signal for you. That's where the Alligator Technique comes in.

First decide that you want to start paying attention to your negative self-talk, that you want to stop it from getting out of hand. Then choose a symbol that will stand out in your mind. (Since they can be dangerous, and since few people like them, we've chosen an alligator, but you can pick any warning symbol that works for you — a red stoplight, a scorpion, a falling boulder — anything that will make you stop and think.) The next time you catch your thoughts running away with you, stop and think "Alligator."

Example:

"Geez, that customer was mad at me. I did everything I could and nothing helped. I just know she's going to complain to my boss. He's going to think I'm really stupid. And incompetent. Wait'll the next time he sees me. He'll probably give me all kinds of grief and ... ALLIGATOR. Wait a minute, wait a minute. Think this over a bit."

The Alligator Technique is a very simple method for cutting off your train of thought before that train runs off the rails. It gives you time to stop and analyze the situation — and your reaction to it — more rationally.

Is there a mental warning symbol that will work for you? Think of one and jot it down below. And the next time your thoughts are racing away with you, stop and shout it to yourself.

____

____

____

LEAP NOT TO CONCLUSIONS

If there were a commandment for keeping your thinking on track, it should probably read, "Leap not to conclusions." When it comes to driving ourselves a little batty with negative thinking, jumping to conclusions — unwarranted conclusions — is often the reason why. We do this in a variety of ways:

1. By distorting or exaggerating parts of the information ("No one said, 'great presentation' to me. No one asked any questions. I blew it big time.")

2. By assuming a complete black-and-white attitude ("If they don't give me the yearly raise, my career here is finished.")

3. By predicting disaster ("If I get fired here, I'll never get another job.")

4. By assuming you know what others will think ("The boss will think I'm an idiot.")

Jumping to unwarranted conclusions is at the heart of many a negative self-talking sequence. And as we said before, it can happen so quickly that sometimes you are barely aware of what you're doing. Memorize these four means of jumping to conclusions so you can stop yourself before you leap.

A FUN EXERCISE TO SEE IF YOU CAN DRIVE YOURSELF BONKERS

Let's see if we can turn some of those negative stress-thinking patterns against themselves by discovering how absurd they can get. Below is a self-talk sequence that starts out logically, but then goes out of control. Read it first. Then in the space below, write a sequence of your own.

Based on your own work experience, create a self-talk pattern you might have thought. Start logically but make each following thought as ridiculous and far out as you can. When you have finished, go over it and put a check mark anywhere you could have used the Alligator Technique for interrupting your thought pattern.

Example:

"I can't believe my presentation didn't get a better response. The client never even thanked me. He must have hated it. They'll never go with our company now, and it'll be my fault. Everyone in the company is going to know. Before long everyone in the industry will know. I blew it and sooner or later they'll let me go. Then what? I'll never get another job. I'll have to do something else with my life. I won't be able to afford my apartment anymore. I'll have to sell my car and get an old clunker. I'll have to take a minimum wage job. I'll probably end up as a bag lady. All because of this one stupid presentation."

Now you try. (Don't be afraid to have a little fun with it.)

By reading over the example and what you have just written, you can see the entire self-talk sequence is absurd.

Which is exactly the point of this exercise.

The self-talk we indulge in can get to the point of absurdity very easily, and it often does. Yet to the person thinking it, it is not that far out at all. By the time we come to our senses, the stress has been created and the damage done. Try to use your version of the Alligator Technique to stop those destructive thought sequences before they can get rolling.

CASE STUDY:
AN ENCOUNTER IN THE ELEVATOR

Leaving work at the end of the day, Sandra dashed into the elevator, where she encountered the manager of the company, a woman Sandra barely knew. Smiling a bit nervously, she pushed the down button. The doors closed and the two of them were alone.

Suddenly, the elevator stalled and came to an abrupt stop between floors.

"Uh-oh," Sandra said, "looks like we have a problem." The manager merely nodded. *Idiot, Sandra thought. Of course we have a problem. What a stupid thing to say.*

"Hope we're not stuck here too long," Sandra said.

"Me too," her boss said. There was a moment's silence.

Dummy, Sandra told herself. Say something intelligent.

"I've been working on the G.Z.T. project like crazy all day and I'm bushed."

"Yes, it's been pretty busy lately, hasn't it?" the manager replied.

You are so stupid, Sandra. Saying you've been working *all day at work. Just brilliant.*

"What do you think we should do?"

Sandra's boss reached forward and pushed the alarm button. A few seconds later the elevator began to move. As the two women walked out, Sandra said, "Oh, I'm Sandra Smith, by the way."

The manager smiled as she left. "Yes, I know. Have a nice night."

Sandra went home mentally kicking herself. The entire evening she worried about the terrible impression she had made on the company manager. "The woman must wonder how in the world I ever got hired," she thought.

What could you tell Sandra about her self-talk? Based on what you've learned in this session, what are some of the errors she made? Some clues are in the *Answers Section* on page 30.

____

____

____

QUIZ

Actions Too Can Bring on a Positive Attitude

With all this talk about self-talk, let's not forget that sometimes actions can indeed speak louder than words. Even if you're having a bad day or when you're feeling down, depressed, or stressed, taking positive actions can actually help lead you to a positive attitude. Here's a chance to see how good you are at turning your attitude around through positive actions. Answer each question **YES** or **NO**; then score yourself below.

	YES	NO
1. Do you arrive at work early enough to plan your day's goals?	______	______
2. Do you answer each phone call with an enthusiastic greeting?	______	______
3. Do you take the time to serve on special committees to help improve the company?	______	______
4. Do you look upon difficult customers as a challenging opportunity to provide more service?	______	______
5. Do you start each day with a heartfelt "Good morning!" to your co-workers?	______	______
6. Are you always aware that to outsiders you contact, you are the company?	______	______
7. Are you willing to make yourself a more valuable employee by spending some time each week learning about your organization's products and services?	______	______
8. Do you avoid those co-workers who spend their time speaking negatively about their work and the company?	______	______
9. Do you make the effort to sound as if you are truly interested in helping customers?	______	______
10. Do you believe you can make a difference?	______	______
Total Number of **YES** Answers	____________	

SCORE YOURSELF: If you scored eight or more **YES** answers, congratulations. You regularly engage in actions that bring a positive attitude to yourself and others. If you scored less, remember that a good attitude will not only reduce your stress level, but it will also help retain customers and keep you in line for bigger and better things.

ANSWERS SECTION

FROM AM I MY OWN WORST ENEMY?

1. He's got to be an idiot to think I can get this done in a week. He should know that isn't possible. Why is he doing this to me?

   You are, in effect, believing that you can read your supervisor's mind. You are assuming that he does not realize the amount of work involved or that you are fairly new on the job. Chances are good that this is untrue. It's very possible that he gave you the project simply because you are new. He has already told you he's looking for some fresh thinking, which supports that conclusion, but you are listening "selectively," that is, you are distorting your thinking by reacting to only part of the incident. Also, you are blaming the boss for giving you the project — a form of negative thinking that rarely gets you anywhere.

2. If I don't come up with the solution, he'll think I'm dumb. How am I supposed to solve the problem when no one else has so far?

   You are predicting the future in a negative fashion. "*If* I don't come up with the solution, he'll think I'm dumb." Others have tried and failed. Your boss knows this. Why should he think you're dumb if you don't come up with the answer? Besides, who is to say that you won't find a workable solution, or at least a partial answer that your manager can use?

   You are also exaggerating the matter by building up the difficulty of the project that, in your mind, gives you an excuse for failing, which you are likely to do with this kind of thinking.

3. If I don't do a great job on this, I'm done for. I'll be back on the street looking for another job in no time.

   This is an example of thinking in black and white. It's either-or with no middle ground. Either you'll do a fantastic job and everything will be great, or it's the end of your world as you know it. Talk about making mountains out of molehills. Try to gain a little perspective on this.

Examples of positive self-talk statements:

1. I guess I should be flattered that he's giving this assignment to me. But one week to do it in? I'm really going to have go all out on it.

2. Wouldn't it be terrific if I could come up with the solution after everybody else here has failed? Talk about making a good first impression.

3. This is going to be a tough nut to crack, but if I fail at least I won't be the first one.

FROM CASE STUDY:
AN ENCOUNTER IN THE ELEVATOR

Being caught off guard by a superior can be an unexpectedly stressful and awkward situation. It can also be an occasion for unacknowledged negative self-talk, as Sandra demonstrated in the example.

Sandra's first error was not being able to recognize the detrimental effect of her inner monologue. Not only was Sandra's self-talk negative in tone, but it was also consistently belittling to herself. In addition, the self-talk continued to snowball as her thoughts progressed.

After making what would generally be considered a benign comment ("looks like we have a problem"), the first word directed at herself was "Idiot." This was followed by self-talk using words such as stupid and dummy. By using these words to describe herself, Sandra set herself up for a no-win situation.

There are two ways Sandra could have handled this incident and come out unscathed. She could have minimized her conversation with the manager by remarking briefly on the elevator stall, not carrying the dialogue any further. If she found her thoughts heading toward negative self-talk she could have used the Alligator Technique. Or, she could have stepped back and observed the situation for what it really was, a temporary inconvenience that was unrelated to her job performance. The latter would have given her the proper perspective for dealing with this minor problem.

DO YOU REMEMBER?

In *Leap Not to Conclusions*, we listed four ways in which people jump to negative and unwarranted conclusions. Can you remember what they were? Write them below.

1. ____

2. ____

3. ____

4. ____

POST-SESSION SKILL LEVEL ASSESSMENT

Based on what you have learned in Session 2, rate yourself again on the following statements. When you are finished, compare your total score to the one you earned at the beginning of this session.

WEAK	AVERAGE	STRONG
1–4 points	5–7 points	8–10 points

I have a good awareness of my own "self-talk."	__________
I understand the importance of self-talk and its effects on me.	__________
I know how to interrupt or stop negative self-talk.	__________
I know of different actions that can help develop a positive attitude.	__________
I recognize how negative thoughts can get out of control.	__________
I know methods for changing negative thoughts.	__________
I am good at not jumping to negative conclusions.	__________
I am good at not exaggerating a bad situation.	__________
I realize how I put stress on myself.	__________
I avoid excessive worrying about work.	__________
TOTAL RATING	__________

WEAK	FAIR	GOOD	STRONG
Under 40	41–55	56–74	75–100

ACTION PLAN

Many of the skills and techniques you have learned in this session are interrelated. Building on your strengths is a good place to start improving your overall abilities, but you can't afford to overlook your weaknesses either.

List below your three best scores (your strengths) and your three lowest scores (your weaknesses) from the ratings on the preceding page.

STRENGTHS	**WEAKNESSES**
1. ______________________	1. ______________________
2. ______________________	2. ______________________
3. ______________________	3. ______________________

Comparing the two lists, can you see any ways in which you can use your strengths to improve your weaknesses? If so, write them down.

____

____

____

____

____

Now reexamine your three biggest weaknesses. Since it's best to work on them one at a time, list them in order. Start with the one you think will be the easiest to improve upon, followed by a more difficult one, and then the most difficult one.

Next to each, set a timetable for concentrating on them (one week, two weeks, and so on):

WEAKNESSES	**TIMETABLE FOR WORKING ON IMPROVEMENT**
1. ______________________	1. ______________________
2. ______________________	2. ______________________
3. ______________________	3. ______________________

Using the ideas and information from this session, list at least one technique you can practice to improve each weakness.

1. ____

2. ____

3. ____

If you cannot determine a technique or course of action you think will be effective, talk to your supervisor about ideas that can be applied to your specific situation.

At the end of the time frame you set for improvement on *all* your weaknesses, look again at the *Post-Session Skill Level Assessment*. Rate yourself once more on all the statements listed. You will probably find improvement not only in your weak areas, but in the others as well.

SUMMARY

When it comes to stress and your reactions to it, this session could have almost been called "You are what you think." Those thoughts, judgments and opinions that are constantly flitting through our minds play such a major role in how much stress we experience that it is all but impossible to underestimate the effects of self-talk.

The major take-aways from this session should be as follows:

1. To become more aware of your thoughts

2. To analyze your thoughts and realize how they are coloring your stress reactions

3. To change the ones that need changing.

It's the third one that's the hardest. But if you can do the first two, you will be well on your way to succeeding at changing your thoughts as well. The techniques and exercises from this session will help if you remember to employ them.

Understanding Your Stress

INTRODUCTION

Stress comes in many forms, guises, and disguises. It's not always easy to pinpoint the real reason for the stress you feel. It can be even harder to discover the real reasons for your reactions to it.

There are a number of possible explanations for that. First, many of us have never stopped to analyze and sort through our feelings regarding the stress in our lives. We have never tried to take it apart in detail to see what it is and what sort of mayhem it is really causing. Second, there are a number of myths and general misconceptions about stress that get in the way of our understanding.

In Session 3, **Understanding Your Stress,** we are going to address both of these issues. We will also try to provide you with workable techniques for controlling the stresses you run into on the job.

We begin with the *Pre-Session Skill Level Assessment*, your self-rating system on your abilities at reducing job stress. Next is *Your Personal 9-Step Stress Examiner,* an exercise designed to help you focus on the causes and possible solutions to the stresses you are having at work.

Our *Quiz: How Well Do You Cope with Stress?* contains many valuable suggestions for doing just that. Then, *A Quick Stress Quiz* will test your knowledge, attitudes, and beliefs regarding stress.

You are probably in for a few surprises when we bring you *Common Myths About Stress,* which is the next feature. We're almost willing to bet that you hold at least one of these widely believed falsehoods.

We begin to move into the realm of methods and techniques for dealing with stress in the next article, *Five Quick Tips for Coping with Stress.* These simple, straightforward tips will get you started on the actions you can take to reduce stress. (Session 4 in its entirety will be devoted to stress-reducing techniques in detail.)

Our *Case Study: Wishing on a Job* will give you a chance to try to figure out how those myths about stress can subtly affect your career in negative ways.

The *Answers Section* will clear up any lingering questions, our *Do You Remember?* quiz will test your memory, and our *Post-Session Skill Level Assessment* will show you how far you've progressed in the minutes spent on this session. The *Action Plan* at the end of the session will help you spot any of your weak areas and give you an approach for developing your skills.

As we said before, stress can be difficult to pin down under the best of circumstances, and you can't combat it if you don't know precisely what you're up against. With that as our goal, we now present Session 3, **Understanding Your Stress.**

PRE-SESSION SKILL LEVEL ASSESSMENT

Using the chart below, rate your own skills as they relate to the following statements.

WEAK	AVERAGE	STRONG
1–4 points	5–7 points	8–10 points

I understand my stressful feelings; I know why I am stressed.	________
I know how to examine my thoughts and feelings on stress.	________
I am good at learning from my thoughts and feelings on stress.	________
I prepare strategies to help deal with stressful situations.	________
I am able to use a team approach in times of heavy stress.	________
I can often make stress work for me.	________
I do not let stress interfere with my productivity.	________
I realize that stress is unavoidable.	________
I am willing to accept stress and deal with it.	________
I understand the difference between internal and external stress.	________
TOTAL RATING	________

WEAK	FAIR	GOOD	STRONG
Under 40	41–55	56–74	75–100

A total score of 55 or less means there is room for improvement. A score between 56 and 74 means you are doing well but can do better. Any score over 75 means it is just a matter of building on your strengths.

YOUR PERSONAL 9-STEP STRESS EXAMINER

We all know what stress is. In fact, we are so familiar with it that we rarely even stop to think about it in any great detail. Stress is stress. We try to avoid it, control it, and deal with it. But we rarely bother to look beneath the surface to see what it is really doing to us and why.

Do you think about stress in your job? Have you ever stopped to really examine it? If you're like most people, you probably haven't.

Here's a chance to examine your personal attitude toward the stress that you are feeling on the job. Think about each of the following questions and then answer as honestly and carefully as you can. There are no right or wrong answers; only an opportunity to discover what is really at the root of some of your workplace stress.

1. If I were to use one word to describe my stress it would be

____

____

2. My usual reaction to stress is

____

____

3. Most of my stress at work is caused by

____

____

4. How long have I been dealing with this (the type of stress from item 3)?

____

____

5. Do I have any specific methods I use to handle it? If so, what are they?

____

____

6. Do I feel I have been generally successful or unsuccessful in dealing with this particular type of stress? In other words, are my methods for dealing with it working? *Describe why you think they are working (or why not).*

____

____

7. Why does that situation (the answer to item 3) bother me more than other stress situations at work?

____

____

8. Does it (the stress situation from item 3) trigger any nagging inner fear within me? Even a little? What is that fear?

____

____

9. Is that fear exaggerated? Is it realistic? Why or why not?

____

____

If you have made it through all nine statements, you should by now have a much better insight to the workings of and reasons behind some of your personal stresses. This is not a cure-all for them, but it can be a very powerful tool in minimizing and overcoming them. Knowing and understanding the enemy is the first step in defeating him. Think about this nine-step examiner and concentrate in particular on the last few statements and answers. Can you think of any steps to take next?

QUIZ

How Well Do You Cope with Stress?

How effective we are at dealing with stress often depends upon our attitudes and opinions about it. These help to determine our reactions, which in turn affect the amount of stress we experience at work. Take the test below to see how your attitudes toward stress affect your ability to cope with it. Answer each statement **TRUE** or **FALSE**; then score yourself below.

	TRUE	FALSE
1. When I encounter a stressful situation at work, I often get annoyed at the person who is causing it.	______	______
2. I worry about being late for work.	______	______
3. I believe that I am better at my job than my co-workers are at theirs.	______	______
4. I feel that I must be "on top of things" at all times.	______	______
5. Stress in other areas of my life affects my job performance.	______	______
6. Talking with my friends about work problems is not going to do anything to reduce the stress I'm under.	______	______
7. I often think about how boring and routine my job is.	______	______
8. I often wish things were better than they are.	______	______
9. I believe stress always has a negative effect on productivity.	______	______
10. Being organized at work does not really help protect you from stress.	______	______
Total Number of **FALSE** Answers	____________	

SCORE YOURSELF: If you checked **FALSE** for nine or more of the statements, your understanding of stress and ability to cope with it appear to be very good. Six to eight **FALSE** answers means you're experiencing more stress than need be, and anything less than that means your attitudes toward stress are causing you stress. Pay particular attention to the rest of this session, where we will further explain some of the statements.

QUIZ

A Quick Stress Quiz

What opinions and attitudes do you have regarding stress? Are they factual or are they untrue? Here's a quick quiz on some common stress-related beliefs.

	YES	NO
The stress I feel is always bad.	______	______
I believe I could control all that stress if I mastered the right stress-reducing techniques.	______	______
Stress has a negative impact on productivity at work.	______	______
Taking time off from work, when you can do it, will always reduce your stress level.	______	______
Hard-driving, aggressive, Type A personalities cannot really change their high-pressure, high-stress natures.	______	______

You will find the answers along with explanations in the section *Common Myths About Stress* in the next feature.

COMMON MYTHS ABOUT STRESS

Despite all the attention paid to workplace stress — and stress in general — many people still cling to certain myths. This can sometimes cause a person to waste his or her time trying to fight a problem that really isn't the problem.

According to clinical psychologist Dr. J.R. Slosar of The Health and Human Services Group in Mission Viejo, California, the following are some of the most common myths about stress.

All Stress Is Bad

Stress can cause depression, anger, and frustration. It can also cause enthusiasm and create energy and excitement. It depends upon the type of stress and the individual's reaction to it.

Stress is everywhere. It's a part of living. And while it can create many problems, stress can also add spice to life. "Life would be pretty boring without it," Dr. Slosar comments.

We Can Always Control Stress

External stress comes from sources over which we have no influence. No matter how well we learn methods for coping, we can never eliminate them. That furious customer who calls out of the blue or the supervisor who got up on the wrong side of bed that morning are stress producers over which we have no control. We can manage our reactions to minimize the stress we feel, often quite successfully. And we can work to avoid putting more *internal* stress on ourselves. But we cannot always control the workings of *external* stress, that which comes to us from outside.

Stress Hurts Productivity at Work

Again it depends upon the type of stress and the individual's reaction to it. A work environment where prolonged or continued stress is the norm may indeed cause productivity to plummet. On the other hand, a rush job that suddenly appears may galvanize a worker to produce more effectively.

In addition, people's reactions to stress vary. Some people seem to need a certain amount of stress to get them moving at top speed. They are the ones who will put off writing a report until the last minute. Others will do that same report as soon as possible, wanting to avoid the stress of waiting until the last minute. The reaction to stress, Dr. Slosar comments, "is a very individual thing."

Time Off Always Helps

Taking some time off work when stressed out is a frequently recommended remedy, and it sometimes does a world of good. Yet it is not a cure-all and its effectiveness depends upon the circumstances. "For example," Dr. Slosar says, "if all your work simply piles up in your absence, you are going to be facing an even more stressful situation when you return." And thinking about that while you're away from work — even if it's just a day or two — is likely to make that time off less than relaxing. Furthermore, it may be that the source of your stress is somewhere other than the office. If it's at home, for instance, the time off may not do you much good.

A Type A Personality Is Permanent

The hard-charging, driven Type A personality is more prone to stress than a less aggressive personality type. But that does not mean the Type A personality must endure a lifetime of high stress, nor that he or she should just accept it by thinking, "Well, it's just the way I am. I'll have to live with it." Changes and modifications in outlook and attitudes can be made which will substantially reduce the amount of stress even a Type A encounters without altering the basic personality type.

Go back to the *Quick Stress Quiz* you filled out previously. They were statements describing some of the myths related to stress. If you answered **NO** to all of them, you are reasonably myth-free when it comes to your beliefs about stress.

Did you miss any? Which ones? If you're like most people, chances are you missed at least one. As you can see, stress can be difficult to pin down, but the management of stress begins with understanding it.

FIVE QUICK TIPS FOR COPING WITH STRESS

Along with the means for identifying common myths about stress, Dr. Slosar offers the following five tips to help manage your daily stress load.

1. Prepare strategies. Everyone knows that it's just a matter of time before that furious customer or co-worker appears. To minimize the stress he or she will cause, be ready. Prepare a strategy beforehand to deal with it. That strategy can be as simple as having a few sentences written down or memorized that you can use to calm the situation.

If you know you will be meeting with a tough customer or an especially difficult colleague, if you know that sooner or later you will have to deal with a customer who is angry because an order was not delivered or didn't function as expected, preparing a strategy is actually easier because you can tailor your prepared remarks to the specific person or problem.

2. A team approach. There are times when your stress load can become especially intense. Whether it is from a job-related source such as an overload of assignments or from a source outside the workplace such as a severe illness or death in the family, your stress load at these times can make it exceptionally difficult for you to perform. Ask your co-workers to help you through the crisis period by temporarily assuming some of your duties or by simply pitching in to assist. Usually, you will be pleasantly surprised by how willingly they'll help.

The teamwork approach is also effective in reducing stress levels when practiced during non-crisis times. Sharing the stress can minimize it for everyone, and assisting one another on an ongoing basis helps to build a friendly and cooperative work environment — which is another stress reducer.

3. Get out. When it's a pressure-packed day, many people eat a sandwich in the office, spend the lunch hour and breaks inside, or simply work straight through. In fact, many people will follow this practice even when the workload is routine and never leave the confines of their office throughout the day.

"Get out," Dr. Slosar emphasizes. "Get out of the office during the day even if it's just for a short break." Go for a walk or a drive on your lunch hour. Get away from the work environment, even if it's only briefly, at least once during the day. The simple change of scene has a rejuvenating effect and gives you time to calm down and recharge your batteries.

4. Focus on breathing. One of the standard physical reactions to stress relates to breathing. When that stressful situation is upon us, our breathing becomes faster and more shallow. This is turn adds to the stress we are already experiencing. And to make matters worse, we are usually unaware of it because we are concentrating on the situation itself.

"Focus on your breathing," Dr. Slosar recommends. A few deep breaths can slow down your body's stress reaction and calm you down. It's a very simple and effective technique. The only trick is remembering to do it. Putting up a handwritten sign or small poster on your wall, desk, or work station can serve as a helpful reminder.

5. Avoid overuse of stimulants. The negative physical effects of stress are increased by stimulants such as caffeine, nicotine, and others. This helps to wear you down all the more. Try to cut back or cut out your use of stimulants during times of stress.

Try to remember these five tips and make them a part of your stress managing efforts.

CASE STUDY: WISHING ON A JOB

Steve had worked as a rep for two years selling and servicing computer peripherals. He had a knack for it and was always in the top five of the 100 reps at the company. Steve worked on commission for sales and service call charges, and even though he was doing exceptionally well, he was unhappy with the stress involved.

"I could have a bad month and make practically nothing," he told himself. "I could have a bad quarter and my job would be in jeopardy. I am so tired of the stress of making quota, of worrying about it all the time. I wish I had a salaried job where I wouldn't have the stress of worrying about how much I'm earning all the time."

Steve got his wish. Another company offered him a similar job, but this one paid a straight salary instead of a commission. He was quite happy with the new position even though he did not make quite as much money as he did before. But as time went by, he became restless and then bored. Oddly enough, he began to experience even more stress than he had before. He started wondering if maybe he shouldn't start looking for another job.

What should Steve do? Why is he feeling stress on the new job? Based on what you have learned in this session, what mistakes would you say Steve is making? Answers are in the *Answers Section* on page 47.

ANSWERS SECTION

FROM CASE STUDY: WISHING ON A JOB

Steve obviously does not understand stress very well and does not realize its effect upon him. He has bought into the myth that all stress is bad, and his reaction (in his first job) is simply to run from it rather than try to manage it. In his case, it appears that the stress of having to make quota was actually a motivator that helped him to succeed.

This becomes apparent by his reaction to his second job. Without the challenge (and stress) of working on commission, he quickly becomes "restless and bored." Extra efforts or additional successes will not bring the immediate rewards of a larger paycheck as they did before. His feelings of frustration are creating stress.

Steve has also bought into the myth that stress always hurts productivity. Actually, however, he is one of those people upon whom a certain amount and type of stress has the opposite effect.

It seems that Steve is so sensitive to stress that he will do nearly anything to avoid it. He has to learn that external stress cannot always be controlled, and he should learn how to manage his own reactions to help control his internal stress, the stress he is putting on himself in his second job.

There is no such thing as a well-paying, stress-free job. For that matter there is no such thing as a stress-free job. If Steve can learn to control some of his inner reactions to stress, he will probably be better off in a commission situation than a straight salary one.

DO YOU REMEMBER?

Can you recall the *5 Quick Tips for Coping with Stress* in this session? See how many you remember and write them below. If you can't get all five, look them up and write in the ones you forgot.

1. ______________________________

2. ______________________________

3. ______________________________

4. ______________________________

5. ______________________________

Remember the *Common Myths About Stress?* How many of those can you recall? List them below. (There were five.)

1. ____________________

2. ____________________

3. ____________________

4. ____________________

5. ____________________

POST-SESSION SKILL LEVEL ASSESSMENT

Based on what you have learned in Session 3, rate yourself again on the following statements. When you are finished, compare your total score to the one you earned at the beginning of this session.

WEAK	AVERAGE	STRONG
1–4 points	5–7 points	8–10 points

I understand my stressful feelings; I know why I am stressed.	______
I know how to examine my thoughts and feelings on stress.	______
I am good at learning from my thoughts and feelings on stress.	______
I prepare strategies to help deal with stressful situations.	______
I am able to use a team approach in times of heavy stress.	______
I can often make stress work for me.	______
I do not let stress interfere with my productivity.	______
I realize that stress is unavoidable.	______
I am willing to accept stress and deal with it.	______
I understand the difference between internal and external stress.	______
TOTAL RATING	______

WEAK	FAIR	GOOD	STRONG
Under 40	41–55	56–74	75–100

A total score of 55 or less means there is room for improvement. A score between 56 and 74 means you are doing well but can do better. Any score over 75 means it is just a matter of building on your strengths.

ACTION PLAN

Many of the skills and techniques you have learned in this session are interrelated. Building on your strengths is a good place to start improving your overall abilities, but you can't afford to overlook your weaknesses either.

List below your three best scores (your strengths) and your three lowest scores (your weaknesses) from the ratings on the preceding page.

STRENGTHS	WEAKNESSES
1. ____________________	1. ____________________
2. ____________________	2. ____________________
3. ____________________	3. ____________________

Comparing the two lists, can you see any ways in which you can use your strengths to improve your weaknesses? If so, write them down.

____

____

____

____

____

Now reexamine your three biggest weaknesses. Since it's best to work on them one at a time, list them in order. Start with the one you think will be the easiest to improve upon, followed by a more difficult one, and then the most difficult one.

Next to each, set a timetable for concentrating on them (one week, two weeks, and so on):

WEAKNESSES	TIMETABLE FOR WORKING ON IMPROVEMENT
1. ____________________	1. ____________________
2. ____________________	2. ____________________
3. ____________________	3. ____________________

Using the ideas and information from this session, list at least one technique you can practice to improve each weakness.

1. ____

2. ____

3. ____

If you cannot determine a technique or course of action you think will be effective, talk to your supervisor about ideas that can be applied to your specific situation.

At the end of the time frame you set for improvement on *all* your weaknesses, look again at the *Post-Session Skill Level Assessment*. Rate yourself once more on all the statements listed. You will probably find improvement not only in your weak areas, but in the others as well.

SUMMARY

One of the main lessons to remember from Session 3 is that there are different kinds of stress. Stress can be positive, negative, or benign; good, bad, or indifferent. Having a baby or even winning the lottery can be highly stressful, but it's a "good" stress. Getting chewed out by the boss or a customer is also highly stressful and, of course, is a "bad" stress. The effects of benign or indifferent stress are a matter of your reaction. The rainstorm that hits at closing time may not mean a thing to you if you remembered your umbrella.

Also remember that you cannot always control stress. You can work to manage and control your internal reactions to it, and thereby reduce the stress level you experience. But to expect to avoid all external stresses is unrealistic. Many times this is beyond your control. All the more reason to work on your reactions to it.

4

Angry Customers & Other Stressful Situations

INTRODUCTION

In Session 4, we are going to begin to explore some of the countermeasures you can employ. We'll be showing you a variety of techniques, approaches, and methods that you can use every day at work to defend yourself against the onset and onslaughts of work-related stress. We'll be explaining what's behind some of these stressful occasions and what you can — and cannot — do to handle them.

We'll focus first on the stress caused by that ever-present problem, the angry customer. In fact, we're going to take it a step further and explore the special problems created by unusually obnoxious or abusive ones. And when we say *customers,* we mean the external customer who buys and uses your company's products or services, and also the internal customer: your boss, a co-worker — anyone who is affected by the performance of your job functions. Every employee has customers. We will also be taking a look at stresses that stem from noncustomer sources such as work overloads, conflicts, and other internal office problems.

Our *Pre-Session Skill Level Assessment* will get you started and give you an idea of what's to come. As before, it will provide you with a benchmark for assessing your own progress.

Did you know that you can actually prepare for stressful situations, even when you don't know when they'll occur? It's true, and we'll show you how in the opening exercise for Session 4, *Prepare for Less Stress*.

The next article will give you valuable advice on dealing with the worst of the worst. It's called *The Nightmare Customer: 5 Steps Toward Defusing High-Stress Situations*. If you have ever had to deal with that type of customer (and who among us hasn't?), you're going to find it particularly informative.

Our session quiz this time is a true-or-false quiz that will test your knowledge of what to say and not to say. It's simply called *Calming Down Angry Customers.*

The following feature will give you additional insights to those nasty customer types and how to deal with the stress they create. You'll find some reassurance, as well, in *A Jerk Is Always a Jerk.*

Moving into the more general realm of office problems, we present *Six More Stress Reducers*, a half dozen handy courses of action you can take to handle a variety of stress-related problems.

After that we'll give you a chance to put what you've learned to work in our *Case Study: Lawn Mower Madness*.

The *Answer Section* and *Do You Remember?* pop quiz are next, followed by the *Post-Session Skill Level Assessment* and our *Action Plan* for you to devise your own personal improvement plan.

That's what is in store for you in Session 4, **Angry Customers & Other Stressful Situations.**

PRE-SESSION SKILL LEVEL ASSESSMENT

Using the chart below, rate your own skills as they relate to the following statements.

WEAK	AVERAGE	STRONG
1–4 points	5–7 points	8–10 points

I realize that one can prepare for some stressful situations.	________
I know how to prepare for certain stressful situations.	________
I am good at clarifying goals; I am rarely confused about what is expected of me at work.	________
I regularly use stress-reducing techniques at work.	________
I am able to defuse high-stress situations.	________
I am good at sticking with a decision and not second guessing myself.	________
I can handle obnoxious or abusive customers well.	________
I avoid saying the wrong thing; I never add "fuel to the fire" with an angry customer.	________
I am good at identifying and setting priorities at work.	________
I am able to prevent tense and stressful situations from escalating.	________
TOTAL RATING	________

WEAK	FAIR	GOOD	STRONG
Under 40	41–55	56–74	75–100

A total score of 55 or less means there is room for improvement. A score between 56 and 74 means you are doing well but can do better. Any score over 75 means it is just a matter of building on your strengths.

PREPARE FOR LESS STRESS

One key method for reducing stress is to prepare for it. That may strike you, at first, as a near impossibility. If you knew when the stress-producing incident was going to happen — and if you knew exactly what it was going to be — you'd be ready for it, right?

Actually, the answer to that is usually no. Many of us consider the unexpected to be something we cannot anticipate. We don't expect the unexpected and so are caught unprepared.

But stop to think about it a moment. You know for a fact that at some point you are going to be confronted by a stressful situation at work. It's just a matter of when and what that situation will be. You can't often predict the "when," but with a little forethought you can frequently predict the general nature of the "what." And if you can predict it, you can prepare for it.

Using your own experience at work as a guideline, complete this exercise. First, think about your job and determine, from the nature of it, what general stressful situation tends to come up the most often. Describe this situation below.

____

____

____

How frequently do you encounter this situation? Daily? Weekly? Monthly? How many times?

____

____

Is this general stressful situation inherent in the job? In other words, does it "come with the territory"?

____

____

If it is a situation you encounter frequently, the answer to the previous question is almost certainly "yes." That means these "unexpected" stressful situations can be expected to happen with regularity. This means you can prepare for them.

Now let's move from the general to the specific.

Recall a recent example of this type of stress-producing incident. Did it involve that angry customer or co-worker? Describe the nature of it, and write what the person said.

____

____

____

Now write, as well as you can remember, how you dealt with it.

____

____

____

With the benefit of hindsight, what could you have said or done that would have been better? What do you wish you had said or done?

____

____

____

What specific incidents, complaint, or complaints cause you the most stress?

____

____

____

Keeping those in mind, prepare for yourself a course of action. Use one of the specific incidents or complaints as a starting point. Then write the statements you can make and any actions you can take to rectify the situation as smoothly as possible. Try to memorize the statements (or keep a copy at your desk) so that you will be prepared the next time this occurs.

Your objective is to have a "script" you can follow to deal with the situation. (You can prepare one for each situation you encounter with some regularity.)

Knowing precisely how you will resolve the problem as it first arises will reduce or eliminate the stress you feel from it.

Example: Your first statement upon hearing the problem: "I'm sorry to hear that. First let me get your name."

First Statement

____

____

Second Statement

____

____

Third Statement

____

____

Additional Statements and/or Actions You Can Take

____

____

____

____

____

____

Save what you have written. Make a copy of it and keep it with you at work until you know it by heart. Over time, take the opportunity to perfect it with any changes that can improve your performance.

THE NIGHTMARE CUSTOMER: 5 STEPS TOWARD DEFUSING HIGH-STRESS SITUATIONS

There will always be times when even the best customers will cause a little stress. But what about the worst of them? Imagine an absolute nightmare of a customer, one who creates a high-stress situation and displays the possibility of actually turning violent if he doesn't get what he wants.

For pointers on dealing with nightmare customers, we can turn to the one profession that deals with the worst nightmare "customers" frequently and regularly — police officers.

What do police officers do to defuse situations? How do they prevent them from escalating? Here are some tips from stress expert and clinical and police psychologist Dr. Hector M. Torres.

1. Listen; don't argue. Arguing with the customer will only inflame the situation — and the customer — all the more. Even when it is blatantly obvious that the customer is wrong, avoid pointing that out or making an issue of it. Now is not the time. Your first objective is to reduce the stress level.

2. Don't defend the company. Defending your company or its policies will automatically tag you as the "opponent" in the customer's mind. It offers the customer an opportunity to focus on you as the embodiment of his anger and frustration. That's the last thing you need.

3. Don't take it personally. This is easier said than done, we know, especially when someone is confronting you. Try to keep in mind that the customer is not screaming at you, Mary Smith, but at the Mary Smith who just happens to be the company's representative at this moment. (All the more reason to pay attention to tip number 2.)

4. Get all the information so you can tell them you're on their side. Ask for all the details, and try to gather all the information you can. This will help in several ways. It allows the customer to get the matter off his chest. (That customer has been waiting, rehearsing in his mind what to say when a listener is finally found. If you don't believe that, think of the last time you were truly teed off.) It also helps lower the tension.

More important, it shows the customer you are really interested and allows you to show that you are going to try to correct matters, that you are on his or her side.

5. Thank them for their patience and understanding. This acknowledges what the customer has been thinking all along: he or she has been imposed upon and unfairly subjected to a major inconvenience. It also compliments the customer, which is a good way of calming that person down.

By using these five tips appropriately, you will usually be able to deescalate the situation, and handle the nightmare customer calmly and efficiently.

QUIZ

Calming Down Angry Customers

Few situations create more stress than having to deal with angry customers. Calming them down will reduce your stress level, of course, but how do you do that? We've already shown you some ways: by trying to support or acknowledge them and by trying to agree with them to defuse their outrage and increase the likelihood of a successful resolution to the problem.

Now let's look at some specific techniques. How do you relieve or moderate a customer's anger and focus the heat away from yourself? How do you help the customer understand that you agree with his or her feelings and are still able to offer a solution? Answer **TRUE** or **FALSE** to the following statements to indicate if they will help you calm down an angry customer and make a sale, overcome an objection, or reach a successful solution.

	TRUE	FALSE
1. I understand most of your concerns.	______	______
2. I know that price is important to your boss.	______	______
3. Once you've had time to think it over, call me.	______	______
4. I'll send you more information immediately.	______	______
5. Aren't you glad I made you aware of that?	______	______
6. I appreciate your feelings about the issue.	______	______
7. I respect your position.	______	______

ANSWERS:

Statement 1: FALSE. This response may make the customer feel as though you don't agree with the details most important to him or her. A better reply would be "I understand your concerns."

Statement 2: FALSE. A reference to the customer's superior may make the matter worse. Try, "I know that price is important to you."

Statement 3: FALSE. If you leave before you settle the issue or agree to the next step, the customer may never call you. Agree with the customer by saying, "Of course you need to think it over. Let's get together early next week to resolve the issue."

Statement 4: TRUE. You may feel that the customer doesn't have all the information needed to make a buying decision. This response implies that the customer will want to know more. It's important to follow up promptly if the meeting ends at this stage.

Statement 5: FALSE. If the customer raises an objection, he or she is not happy about the information. A more professional reply would be, "I'm sorry that information upset you. What bothers you about it?"

Statement 6: TRUE. This is a simple response that merely offers agreement.

Statement 7: TRUE. This reply will help defuse the situation as long as you sincerely feel that way.

Key Point: Shifting a customer's anger away from you is a smart move. Learn how to defuse a potentially disagreeable situation and you will minimize the stress.

A JERK IS ALWAYS A JERK

Fortunately the jerks are fairly rare, but not so rare that you will not encounter one from time to time. We're talking about the truly obnoxious co-worker or customer who almost seems to delight in creating stressful and troublesome situations. What can you do about the stress brought on by these people?

"Realize that you can't change these people," says Dr. Torres. "A jerk is always a jerk. They're consistent."

These troublemaking people will behave boorishly with almost anyone, most of the time. Their behavior is not limited to or directed at you in particular. They act that way toward everyone.

What can you do? "If it's justified," Dr. Torres says, "acknowledge the problem and offer to help."

If you find yourself stressing out over them, try to indulge yourself in a bit of mental imagery. In your mind, picture them "with a Mickey Mouse hat or a propeller beanie on." This can help cut them down to size in your mind and put them in an entirely new, lower stress category. Another solution, again, is to do your best to not take the abuse personally.

SIX MORE STRESS REDUCERS

Stress can be caused by all manner of things: work overload, moving into new areas of responsibility, and unclear directions from supervisors — to name just a few.

Following are descriptions of some common stress-producing work situations, along with a number of actions you can take to address the problem. Match the actions to the situations as indicated. Answers are in the *Answers Section* on page 65.

Actions

A. Identify priorities. Separate the wheat from the chaff. Make a list of all the tasks you have to accomplish and rank them in order of importance. Then deal with them in that order.

B. Get organized. Keep ongoing projects updated. Have all the items necessary for your job on hand at all times. Schedule your workday, insofar as it is possible, in order to manage your time better. Set aside a specific time each day to handle the unexpected tasks that always crop up.

C. Get regular physical exercise. What you have always been told is true. One of the best antidotes to stress is a program of regular physical exercise. At the very least, see to it that you exercise whenever you can, even if it is only a matter of taking a daily walk.

D. Clarify goals. It's difficult to do a good job when you're not completely sure what your job is. Unclear goals in your job description are a sign of a lack of direction from management; it's a situation that sometimes goes on for extended periods of time. Ask your supervisors to clarify them for you. If they cannot, ask specifically what they expect from you.

E. Don't waffle. Once you have made a decision, stick with it. If you have determined a course of action, pursue it. Don't waste time and energy second-guessing yourself. Worrying about making a decision can be stressful enough. Going over the same ground again, making and remaking that decision, can bring on a tremendous amount of stress.

F. Take a break. It's another well-worn piece of advice, but it's one that constantly bears repeating. When stress starts to overwhelm you, take a break. Often 10 or 15 minutes away is all you need to get back on an even keel.

Stress Situations

1. Things are going fine when suddenly three pesky problems hit at the same time. All of them have to be resolved today, all are equally important, and you hardly know where to start.

   Action Letter ____

2. Each day at work seems to be frantic. You're always busy and seem to be running all day just to stay in place. You usually have to stay late to catch up.

   Action Letter ____

3. You have a predetermined number of calls to make each day, and there is usually just enough time to make them. Now your supervisor wants you to take on another responsibility and do a little selling over the phone as well. It's a new area for you, and you are uneasy about it.

   Action Letter ____

4. Over the past months, the pace at work seems to have slowly increased. You find yourself getting tired, irritable and short-tempered. Even when you finish everything by five, you worry about work in the evening and are worn out long before bedtime.

   Action Letter ____

5. Your supervisor has given you a special project, hinting that it could be a prelude to a raise and promotion. She expects you to do it in addition to your regular duties. You quickly determine that there isn't enough time to do both jobs well. You want to meet with her to explain the situation, but you don't want to take the chance of blowing a promotion opportunity.

   Action Letter ____

6. You find it difficult at work to determine which projects should command the majority of your attention. Every time you concentrate on one, it seems that another turns out to be more important. You are constantly dropping one project to rush to another.

   Action Letter ____

CASE STUDY: LAWN MOWER MADNESS

The problem is clearly the customer's fault. One look at the lawn mower he bought from your company is enough to show you that he assembled it incorrectly. Normally, you'd apologize for his inconvenience and have it reassembled for him. But that's not enough for this guy.

He's shouting at you, feeding on his own fury, and growing angrier by the minute. You feel like you're walking on eggs. If you're not very careful in what you say or do, it seems to you that he's likely to explode. And, truth be told, you're a little intimidated. You're a good customer service rep; you know how to handle tough customers. Even furious ones. But this guy is something else. He's on the verge of turning physically violent, and you haven't been trained to handle anything like this. Now what do you do?

Suggested approaches are in the *Answers Section* on page 65.

ANSWERS SECTION

FROM SIX MORE STRESS REDUCERS

Stress Situation	Action
1	F
2	B
3	D
4	C
5	E
6	A

FROM CASE STUDY: LAWN MOWER MADNESS

In *The Nightmare Customer* we listed five steps for defusing high-stress situations. This situation certainly falls in that category, and those are the procedures to follow in order to deal with the customer in the case study. How many of those five steps did you employ in your answer? Look back to page 59 to find out.

DO YOU REMEMBER?

Can you recall the stress-reducing actions you could take that were covered in *Six More Stress Reducers*? Write them below.

1. ____

2. ____

3. ____

4. ____

5. ____

6. ____

POST-SESSION SKILL LEVEL ASSESSMENT

Based on what you have learned in Session 4, rate yourself again on the following statements. When you are finished, compare your total score to the one you earned at the beginning of this session.

WEAK	AVERAGE	STRONG
1–4 points	5–7 points	8–10 points

I realize that one can prepare for some stressful situations. __________

I know how to prepare for certain stressful situations. __________

I am good at clarifying goals; I am rarely confused about what is expected of me at work. __________

I regularly use stress-reducing techniques at work. __________

I am able to defuse high-stress situations. __________

I am good at sticking with a decision and not second guessing myself. __________

I can handle obnoxious or abusive customers well. __________

I avoid saying the wrong thing; I never add "fuel to the fire" with an angry customer. __________

I am good at identifying and setting priorities at work. __________

I am able to prevent tense and stressful situations from escalating. __________

TOTAL RATING __________

WEAK	FAIR	GOOD	STRONG
Under 40	41–55	56–74	75–100

A total score of 55 or less means there is room for improvement. A score between 56 and 74 means you are doing well but can do better. Any score over 75 means it is just a matter of building on your strengths.

ACTION PLAN

Many of the skills and techniques you have learned in this session are interrelated. Building on your strengths is a good place to start improving your overall abilities, but you can't afford to overlook your weaknesses either.

List below your three best scores (your strengths) and your three lowest scores (your weaknesses) from the ratings on the preceding page.

STRENGTHS	**WEAKNESSES**
1. ____________________	1. ____________________
2. ____________________	2. ____________________
3. ____________________	3. ____________________

Comparing the two lists, can you see any ways in which you can use your strengths to improve your weaknesses? If so, write them down.

____

____

____

____

____

Now reexamine your three biggest weaknesses. Since it's best to work on them one at a time, list them in order. Start with the one you think will be the easiest to improve upon, followed by a more difficult one, and then the most difficult one.

Next to each, set a timetable for concentrating on them (one week, two weeks, and so on):

WEAKNESSES	**TIMETABLE FOR WORKING ON IMPROVEMENT**
1. ____________________	1. ____________________
2. ____________________	2. ____________________
3. ____________________	3. ____________________

Using the ideas and information from this session, list at least one technique you can practice to improve each weakness.

1. ____

2. ____

3. ____

If you cannot determine a technique or course of action you think will be effective, talk to your supervisor about ideas that can be applied to your specific situation.

At the end of the time frame you set for improvement on *all* your weaknesses, look again at the *Post-Session Skill Level Assessment*. Rate yourself once more on all the statements listed. You will probably find improvement not only in your weak areas, but in the others as well.

SUMMARY

There is no getting around the fact that you will encounter angry or rude customers or co-workers throughout your career. They can cause you a great deal of stress, or you can minimize and even eliminate their ability to affect you. The methods in this session have shown you some ways to accomplish that. Knowing that this will inevitably happen at some time or other, you can be prepared.

Another key lesson from this session involves the continual stress you feel. Whether it's the structure of your company, your job description (or lack thereof), or conflicts with co-workers or superiors, put the stress reducers into practice. You will find the quality of your work life will improve as your ability to deal with those stresses improves.

5

Humor & Crisis: The Light and Dark Sides of Stress

INTRODUCTION

Session 5 is roughly divided into two parts.

In the first part we'll continue to look at more strategies and techniques for managing and controlling stress. As serious and effective as some of them can be, we think you'll find it a somewhat lighthearted approach to the problem, and we think it's highly appropriate. After all, if stress has one single deadly enemy, it is laughter.

The second part of Session 5 is about as serious as stress can get. It deals with an end result of prolonged stress — namely burnout. This tragedy can be avoided, even for someone already in its early stages.

After our *Pre-Session Skill Level Assessment*, Session 5 gets going with *"Don't Take It Personally???" Oh, Sure*, a wry look at why it is so difficult not to take all those stress-building insults and affronts personally.

Have you ever imagined that mean, huge, hulking, stress-producing person in a ballet tutu? What's going on here? It's *Mental Imaging*, a fun technique for lowering your stress by changing your attitude toward its source.

Likewise, do you ever try to stay angry, tense, or upset when you're laughing? It's all but impossible, which may be why laughter is one of the best stress relievers going. Helping you shore up this stress defense is not (or is it?) a laughing matter, which is why we present *Humor: The Great Antidote,* followed by *Five Tips to Develop Your Humor.*

Our *Quiz: Say Yes to Sometimes Saying No* tracks your ability to keep from being overwhelmed at work simply because you're a nice person. There are times when you have to be extra assertive, and this quiz will help determine if you are.

Then we turn to the serious side with *Burnout, Part I: Warning Signs.* Knowing what to look for in yourself and others is the first step toward recognizing that this complex phenomenon is actually occurring.

Burnout, Part II: Pouring Water on the Fire will show you how to counteract the stress that leads to burnout, even when the process is already under way.

Our *Case Study: The Fine Art of Saying No* will give you an opportunity to figure out a thorny, stress-related problem and the chance to brush up on your "saying no" skills as well.

Our *Answers* and *Do You Remember?* sections follow, and this last session is also concluded with our *Post-Session Skill Level Assessment* and *Action Plan* features.

It's all ahead in the fifth and final session, **Humor & Crisis: The Light and Dark Sides of Stress.**

PRE-SESSION SKILL LEVEL ASSESSMENT

Using the chart below, rate your own skills as they relate to the following statements.

WEAK	AVERAGE	STRONG
1–4 points	5–7 points	8–10 points

I don't let rude or angry customers/co-workers get to me.	_______
I know how to use mental imaging to reduce stress.	_______
I maintain and display a sense of humor on the job.	_______
I often look for and find the humor in tough situations.	_______
I am fairly assertive about saying no to requests when necessary.	_______
I know what "burnout" and its consequences are.	_______
I can recognize some of the signs of imminent burnout.	_______
I am good at diplomatically saying no.	_______
I am able to express my emotions when under heavy stress.	_______
I realize the role physical activity plays in reducing stress.	_______
TOTAL RATING	_______

WEAK	FAIR	GOOD	STRONG
Under 40	41–55	56–74	75–100

A total score of 55 or less means there is room for improvement. A score between 56 and 74 means you are doing well but can do better. Any score over 75 means it is just a matter of building on your strengths.

"DON'T TAKE IT PERSONALLY???" OH, SURE.

On a couple of occasions in this workbook, when explaining how to handle the stress of dealing with angry people, we have pointed out that the anger or criticism is not directed at you personally. Keeping that in mind is a good way to limit your reactions to it, in effect, to shrug it off. "Don't take it personally" the admonition goes, and it is, in fact, a solid piece of advice for managing stress.

Except …

We can't help being reminded of a scene that pops up in one form or another in many a gangster or Mafia movies. The head bad guy has cornered his opponent and is about to do him in for good. He pauses and says something along the lines of, "I want you to know there's nothing personal in this, Vince. It's just business."

And then … *bang, bang, bang*. That's the end of poor Vince, who was no doubt vastly relieved that there was nothing personal in his getting shot to death. On the other hand, he may have wondered, however briefly, "Personal, business, what's the difference?" and may have found it just a wee bit difficult not to take it all very personally indeed.

When someone is taking out all his or her anger on you, it's hard not to take it personally, at least in part. When someone is yelling and screaming at you, or being snidely sarcastic at your expense, you would have to be a saint or an emotionless automaton not to take some offense. It's human nature.

With practice and enough experience, you may learn the ability to shrug it off so that you do not feel any of the accompanying stress. In order to help you reach that point, we're going to suggest the following technique as one way to accomplish it. The next time someone is raising your stress level up to the 101st Airborne Division parachute altitude, try a little mental imagery. We have touched on this method before, and here's how to make it work for you.

M E N T A L   I M A G I N G

Picture that person in a ridiculous setting. (We mentioned picturing the "jerk" in a Mickey Mouse hat or propeller beanie in Session 4.) The mental image of this obnoxious customer suddenly looking silly has a way of cutting that person down to size in your thoughts and reactions. It's difficult to feel fearful, intimidated, or stressful when you're secretly minimizing, even laughing at, the source of the stress. Mental imagery can help you do that.

Do the following exercise. Make a list of mental images you can create for obnoxious and unruly people. Build those images around something you find humorous or amusing. Write them below. (You may find it useful to create separate images for males and females.) When you are finished, take a few moments to memorize those images so you can readily picture them in your mind when the next occasion arises.

To begin, write:

I picture this person wearing ... or ...

I picture this person dressed in ... or ...

I picture this person in a ...

1. ______________________________

2. ______________________________

3. ______________________________

4. ______________________________

Now try the same thing for the difficult people who cause you stress whom you know — that is, co-workers, customers, clients, or others you deal with on an ongoing basis, as opposed to unknown and unseen callers. This will be just a little harder, but potentially more useful. (Helpful hint: If that person is a supervisor or co-worker who may be in the same room with you now, don't write the person's name, or if you must, do it in code.)

1. ______________________________

2. ______________________________

3. ______________________________

4. ______________________________

Picture this: The next time one of these people is a source of stress for you, imagine him or her like this. And don't take it personally.

HUMOR: THE GREAT ANTIDOTE

What characteristic do you look for most in your friends? Certainly near the top of almost everyone's list would be a sense of humor. Everyone likes humor and the opportunity to enjoy a hearty laugh. Yet for some mysterious reason, many of us leave humor at the door when we come to work each day. "Most of us are far too serious," declares consultant Terry L. Paulson, Ph.D. "U.S. workers consume over 15 *tons* of aspirin a day. We move steadily through life with flat expressions on our faces. We've lost touch with the importance of fun in the workplace."

Human beings by nature are playful and spontaneous creatures. "We get 'professionally' serious and then pay comedians to do a job we've forgotten to do ourselves," muses Paulson. "Most of us were trained to put a lid on our humor, but we still tend to respect people who use it. People with a sense of humor are people you want to work with and listen to, and whose products you want to buy," he says.

Customers appreciate humor. Customer service is serious business, but a tactful dash of humor can help resolve difficult situations — and help keep customers satisfied at the same time. That's what happened when a customer came into a bank fuming over an error. As he approached the teller's window, however, he saw a small sign: "Mistakes made while you wait." The customer smiled, then chuckled. His anger dissipated, and he explained the problem without rancor. The teller apologized for the problem and quickly corrected it.

Humor is good for you, too. It can help you relax, release tension and anger, and put you in a better mood. In short, humor — and the laughter it brings — is a great antidote to stress.

5 TIPS TO DEVELOP YOUR HUMOR

"One of the best ways to fight on-the-job stress is with a good laugh," says Dr. Joel Goodman, consultant and director of The HUMOR Project, Inc., in Saratoga Springs, New York. "Take your job seriously and yourself lightly," says Goodman. He offers the following five tips:

1. Tell yourself, "At least I'll get a good story out of this," and anticipate telling it. Some companies even have regular sessions in which employees share experiences and reward the best storyteller. And, of course, friends and co-workers always like to hear an amusing anecdote.

2. Post a humorous quote in your work area. You might also put a quote on a placard, change it weekly, and let customers see it.

3. Enhance relationships. Humorist Victor Borge once said, "A smile is the shortest distance between two people." Smiles help build relationships. "People often mirror what they see or sense," says Goodman. "If you smile, even on the phone, you increase the likelihood that others will smile, too."

4. Increase creativity. Ask yourself how your favorite comedian would see a situation. Encourage a childlike perspective. "When handling a problem, ask yourself, 'How would an 8-year-old see this?'" says Goodman. "Your answers … can make you laugh internally and change your perspective."

5. Laugh with — not at — people. Use humor as a tool to build people up rather than as a weapon to tear them down. Laughing at people creates adversarial relationships. If the humor is demeaning or in bad taste, don't use it.

"You don't have to be a stand-up comedian rattling off one-liners to bring a humorous outlook to your job," Goodman says. "A simple smile or inviting lightness by asking customers to share their own humor can be major steps."

How can you put more humor into your workplace? Putting these five tips into action can help. What else can you do? Well, you tell us. Write a few of your own ideas below.

1. ______________________________

2. ______________________________

3. ______________________________

4. ______________________________

QUIZ

Say Yes to Sometimes Saying No

Sometimes, for your own well-being, it's important to know when to pull in the reins a bit and say no. Sometimes you have to be a little assertive in order to protect yourself from a stress overload caused by trying to do too much work or by trying to please too many people too much of the time. And sometimes the requests made of you, even by the boss, can be very unreasonable.

Are you stressing yourself out by being too eager to please? Take the following test and find out. Answer each question **YES** or **NO**; then score yourself below.

	YES	NO
1. Do you say yes to impossible requests just so you won't offend others?	______	______
2. Do you think your job requires you to always say yes?	______	______
3. Do you say yes out of fear that customers will never do business with you again?	______	______
4. Do you say yes because you think you are the only person who can handle the request?	______	______
5. Do you say yes to every request from co-workers?	______	______
6. Do you say yes to all requests from your supervisor, even if the request is impossible to carry out?	______	______
7. Do you feel you must help everyone, regardless of the importance of his or her request?	______	______
8. Do you say yes because it's easier than saying no?	______	______
9. Does saying yes to everyone you work with make you feel needed?	______	______
10. Do you say yes because you feel guilty when you say no?	______	______
Total Number of **YES** Answers	____________	

SCORE YOURSELF: Fewer than three **YES** answers indicates you're able to say no to requests that have little to do with effective service. If you scored more than three **YES** answers, you need to examine why you have trouble saying no. Keep in mind that you can spread yourself too thin by offering help each time someone puts a request before you. When this occurs, you aren't serving anyone effectively. Realize that it's OK to say no sometimes. In fact, sometimes it's better not to say yes.

BURNOUT, PART I: WARNING SIGNS

We all know the results of burnout: loss of interest in the job, poor performance at work, and physical and emotional exhaustion — to name just a few. Yet that is not necessarily the end of it. "Left untreated," says stress expert Dr. Michael B. Pons, "burnout will eventually lead to major medical problems. A heart attack, an ulcer ... it will manifest itself physically in some way."

Burnout itself is the result of prolonged and overwhelming stress. Fortunately, burnout does have its warning signs. The most significant of them, says Dr. Pons, is that the performance level slips. "The person begins missing deadlines, missing appointments. There will be an overall decline in efficiency, a loss of interest and a lack of initiative."

There are other indications of approaching burnout that you can look for as well. But one of the major problems, Pons says, "is that the person who is burning out doesn't realize [it]. It's safe to say that 90% of the people burning out don't recognize that it's happening." And that occurs in spite of the many warning signs they may already be experiencing.

Have you ever worked with someone you thought might be on the verge of burning out? Have you ever felt you might be? Write down what you think are some of the signs and symptoms of burnout. A list of them can be found in the *Answers Section* on page 83.

BURNOUT, PART II: POURING WATER ON THE FIRE

As we said before, most people who are beginning to experience burnout don't realize it. Usually it takes someone else to confront that person with the facts. At that point, the majority do recognize the dilemma.

What then? How do you pour water on the fire? The goal is to control and manage the cause of the threatened burnout: stress. According to Dr. Pons, "it is crucial to be able to express your emotions to others." The simple act of sharing and communicating your concerns with others has a way of dissipating stress.

There are many recommended methods for reducing the stress that can cause burnout, including all of the ones previously covered in this workbook. Here are a few more:

1. Establish a support (buddy) system. It's good to have a mate or a close friend to share your feelings with, but that may not be enough. Dr. Pons suggests that it's better to find a "peer," someone you can talk to who "understands the nature of your work," such as a co-worker at the company, a friend in the same line of business at another company, or someone else who is familiar with the type of work you do.

2. Learn when to say no. Your time and energy are finite. You cannot agree to every request for assistance and to every additional assignment, as much as you might feel you *should*. Agreeing to take on an extra responsibility when you really don't want to will leave you feeling put-upon and can breed anger and hostility. It also puts much more pressure on you to do even more work.

3. Don't feel guilty about saying no. When you are already under a great deal of stress from your own workload (or for other reasons), there is nothing wrong with saying no. Allowing yourself to feel guilty about it will just add more stress despite the fact that you turned down the extra work.

4. If possible, delegate. If it is an option, don't hesitate to delegate some of the workload. If it is not, you can ask a co-worker to help you or talk to your supervisor to request assistance.

5. Talk to your superior. For an ongoing high-stress problem (as opposed to the temporary crunches that come and go in any occupation), the support of your boss will be key to reducing your stress. As a matter of fact, higher management may be a major source of that stress, owing to unrealistic or impractical goals they have set or to responsibilities they have not defined clearly.

6. Avoid back-to-back high-stress situations; plan your day. If and whenever possible, schedule your day to intersperse the high-pressure tasks with the low-pressure ones. For example, if you have two presentations to make that day, avoid scheduling them back to back. Have one in the morning; then give yourself an hour or two to work on a less intense task. Then schedule the second one for the afternoon. This gives you a chance to recharge your batteries.

7. Work physical activity into your routine. The better your physical condition, the better your body is able to withstand stress. Taking part in physical activities is also a terrific way to work off stress. Whether after work, in the morning, or on the lunch hour, engage in a physical activity you enjoy. It is one of the most effective means of combating stress.

CASE STUDY:
THE FINE ART OF SAYING NO

Jim dashed into the office that morning feeling tired already. He was running late despite the fact that he had wanted to get in early to attack the mountain of work awaiting him. Somehow he hadn't made it, and somehow he felt that no matter how hard he worked, the "mountain" wouldn't be any smaller at day's end. Things had been going this way for months, and Jim was beginning to wonder if it was all worth it.

He was expecting an important client to call first thing in the morning. He hoped he hadn't missed the call. Rushing down the hall to his office, he passed the Director of Human Resources. "Jim," she said, "I'd like to have you on the committee for the company's annual charity fund-raiser. Would you give me a call when you have a minute?"

Nodding in agreement, Jim hurried on. As he passed his supervisor's office, he heard the boss call out, "Jim! That new business pitch I mentioned is on. I want you in on it. Stop by as soon as you can."

As he reached his office, one of his co-workers approached him. "Jim, I've got to get all those sales projections done by five, and there's just no way. Can you help me out, please? Just with a few of them?"

The phone in his office rang and Jim grabbed it. He talked with his client for twenty minutes and suggested a solution to the client's rather urgent problem. The client liked Jim's idea and now he had to get it into motion immediately. It would take him the better part of the morning, but at least things were off to a good start. Now he had to deal with the three latest requests.

Jim didn't like serving on committees and did not want to work on the fund-raiser. But the Director of Human Resources had been the person most responsible for hiring him four short months ago.

Jim would like to help out his co-worker — the person had done favors for him in the past — but he just didn't see how he could make the time.

Jim very much wanted to work on the high-profile new business pitch, but again, time was the problem. He is already overburdened and stressed out.

It's pretty obvious *what* Jim should say to two of the requests. But *how* should he say it diplomatically? As for his superior's request that might be more complicated, what would you say? And how would you say it?

Write *how* you would phrase your answers to each of the three requests. There are no right or wrong answers, but in the case of the boss's request, there is an opportunity if you're smart enough to spot it. The answer to that is in the *Answers Section* on page 84.

ANSWERS SECTION

FROM BURNOUT, PART I

The following are among the warning signs of burnout:

1. Low self-esteem
2. Feeling tired, even after getting a good night's sleep
3. Feelings of hostility toward the job
4. Working longer hours, but performance level still declines
5. Very quick to get angry over little things
6. Displaying a certain cynicism or negativism about the job
7. Tendency to be very inflexible
8. Becoming highly irritable
9. Noticeable mood swings
10. Frequent fatigue and weariness
11. Avoiding work or work responsibilities
12. Loss of interest in co-workers/more conflicts with co-workers

This is not a complete list of all the possible warning signs of burnout, just of some of the most common. It should also be emphasized that if someone displays one or two of the signs, it does not necessarily indicate that person is on the edge of burnout. Many of us display some of these attributes at one time or another.

FROM CASE STUDY: THE FINE ART OF SAYING NO

Jim has an opportunity to alleviate his work overload and reduce the stress it is bringing. Because he wants to work on the new business pitch, and because his boss wants him in on it, it makes sense for Jim to agree. His current workload, however, clearly makes that impossible. Jim is already exhibiting a few early signs of burnout.

The boss, however, will expect Jim to put in extra hours to do the new business pitch and might construe Jim's refusal to join as a refusal to work longer or as an inability to get the job done. Jim doesn't want him thinking that he is not willing to work extra hours or is incompetent. Simply pleading that he is already overburdened and saying no in this situation is therefore a risky proposition.

But if Jim shows enthusiasm for working on it (an enthusiasm he does feel), he can raise the issue of his overwork by combining it with another element. In other words, Jim could say, "I'd really love to work on it, but I'm already up to my eyebrows in work and most of my projects can't be put aside. What I'm afraid of is that the *quality* of the work will suffer if I don't have the time to really dig into it. And that's not fair to me, the company, or anybody."

At that point, the boss may suggest a solution (or if he doesn't, Jim could raise the issue) of shifting some of the work to someone else or of giving Jim some temporary help. The key here is that the impetus came from the boss. He wants Jim on the project and Jim is only too willing to help — if the boss can help him out in return. Appealing to their mutual desire to do a first-rate, quality job on the new business pitch is more likely to bring Jim this help than to simply say he is already overworked. Additionally, it opens the door for Jim to talk to the boss again about his stress load farther down the line.

DO YOU REMEMBER?

How many of the *5 Tips to Develop Your Humor* can you recall? Write them below.

1. ______________________________

2. ______________________________

3. ______________________________

4. ______________________________

5. ______________________________

POST-SESSION SKILL LEVEL ASSESSMENT

Based on what you have learned in Session 5, rate yourself again on the following statements. When you are finished, compare your total score to the one you earned at the beginning of this session.

WEAK	AVERAGE	STRONG
1–4 points	5–7 points	8–10 points

I don't let rude or angry customers/co-workers get to me.	______
I know how to use mental imaging to reduce stress.	______
I maintain and display a sense of humor on the job.	______
I often look for and find the humor in tough situations.	______
I am fairly assertive about saying no to requests when necessary.	______
I know what "burnout" and its consequences are.	______
I can recognize some of the signs of imminent burnout.	______
I am good at diplomatically saying no.	______
I am able to express my emotions when under heavy stress.	______
I realize the role physical activity plays in reducing stress.	______
TOTAL RATING	______

WEAK	FAIR	GOOD	STRONG
Under 40	41–55	56–74	75–100

A total score of 55 or less means there is room for improvement. A score between 56 and 74 means you are doing well but can do better. Any score over 75 means it is just a matter of building on your strengths.

ACTION PLAN

Many of the skills and techniques you have learned in this session are interrelated. Building on your strengths is a good place to start improving your overall abilities, but you can't afford to overlook your weaknesses either.

List below your three best scores (your strengths) and your three lowest scores (your weaknesses) from the ratings on the preceding page.

STRENGTHS	**WEAKNESSES**
1. ______________________	1. ______________________
2. ______________________	2. ______________________
3. ______________________	3. ______________________

Comparing the two lists, can you see any ways in which you can use your strengths to improve your weaknesses? If so, write them down.

____

____

____

____

____

Now reexamine your three biggest weaknesses. Since it's best to work on them one at a time, list them in order. Start with the one you think will be the easiest to improve upon, followed by a more difficult one, and then the most difficult one.

Next to each, set a timetable for concentrating on them (one week, two weeks, and so on):

WEAKNESSES	**TIMETABLE FOR WORKING ON IMPROVEMENT**
1. ______________________	1. ______________________
2. ______________________	2. ______________________
3. ______________________	3. ______________________

Using the ideas and information from this session, list at least one technique you can practice to improve each weakness.

1. ____

2. ____

3. ____

If you cannot determine a technique or course of action you think will be effective, talk to your supervisor about ideas that can be applied to your specific situation.

At the end of the time frame you set for improvement on *all* your weaknesses, look again at the *Post-Session Skill Level Assessment.* Rate yourself once more on all the statements listed. You will probably find improvement not only in your weak areas, but in the others as well.

SUMMARY

Learning when and how to say no can save you from a world of stress. You can't please all the people all the time even though you might want to. Stretching yourself to the breaking point does no one any good. Don't be afraid of being a little assertive sometimes. It can be a very necessary act of self-protection.

Finally, the last major lesson from this workbook is one to keep in mind all the time. To put it in terms of a common phrase, "lighten up." You can and should be serious about your job and your career. But there's a big difference between being deadly serious about the job and deadly serious *on* the job. Almost everyone can afford to be a little less serious about him or herself. Everyone likes a cheerful person, and that includes superiors and supervisors as well as clients and customers. A little humor in your outlook helps to keep everything in perspective and helps you to get the best of stress.